ONE MINUTE HEALING

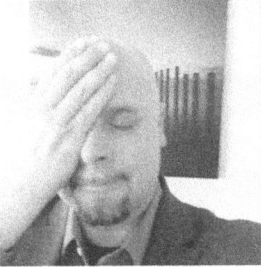

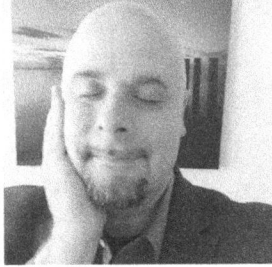

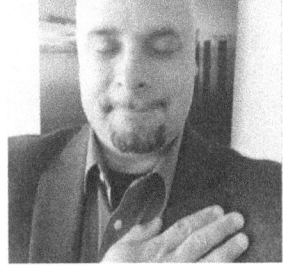

The "PAWS" 🐾 Distress Relief technique, alleviating <u>P</u>ain, <u>A</u>nger, <u>W</u>orry, & <u>S</u>adness * A Complete Guide

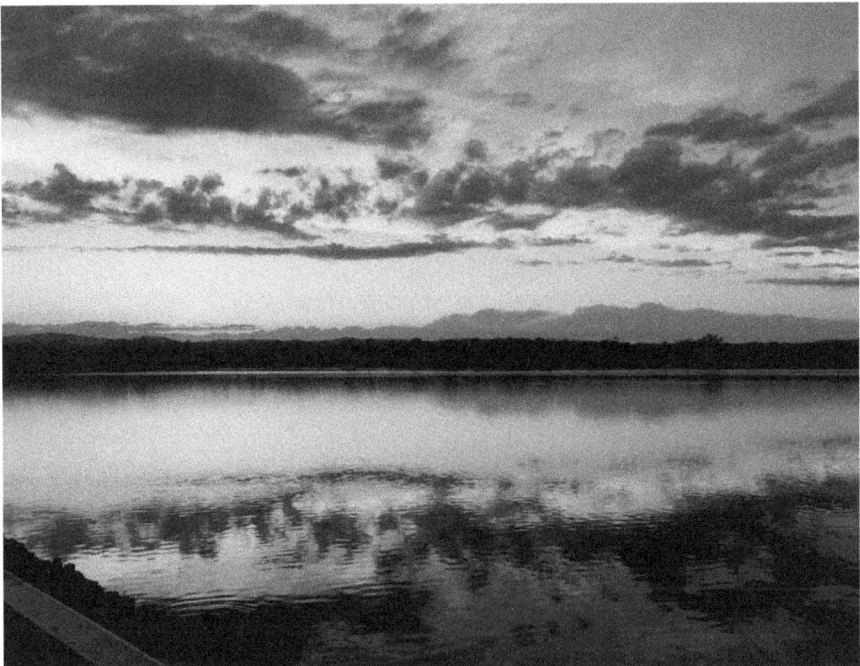

🐾 BY R. WOLF SHIPON, PHD 🐾

ALTERNATIVE HEALING RESEARCHER AND LICENSED PSYCHOLOGIST
REIKI MASTER, CERTIFIED NLP BRIEF THERAPIST & CLINICAL HYPNOTHERAPIST

Dedication

To all the healers out there — especially those who do not know they are healers — such as my wife Jennifer, my son Leo, my family on both sides, all the friends (human and animal) I have ever had, and you.

Table of Contents

Cheat sheet: The PAWS 🐾
Healing System

This healing system reduces the impact of any problem by reducing stress.

STEP ONE: PAWS 1

FIRST PAIN ANGER WORRY SADNESS MEASUREMENT (PAWS Pre-test).

State the problem (Pain, Anger, Worry, or Sadness — PAWS for short, which sounds like *exactly what you need to do* [pause] when you feel these feelings) out loud & rate your distress about the feelings from 0 (best) to 10 (worst).

Raise your eyebrows 3 times, then smile (even forced — fake it until you make it)!

Deep breath in, and slowly exhale.

STEP TWO: USE YOUR PAW! 🐾

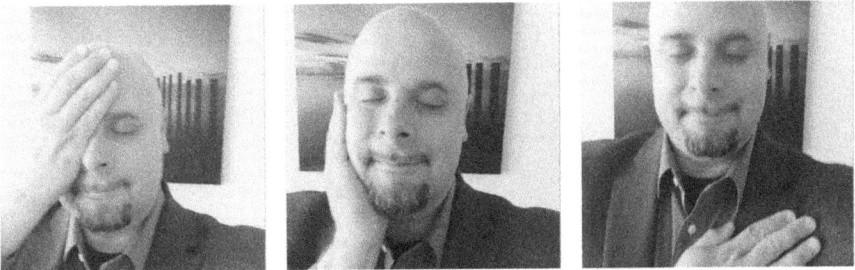

Note: Eyes may be open or closed. This guy likes his eyes closed.

1. Right palm over right eye, paw-like fingers of right hand (held together) on forehead, and say out loud one thing for which you're deeply grateful right now or in the past

2. Paw-like right hand on right side of face, say outloud a second thing for which you're deeply grateful right now or in the past.

3. Paw-like hand over heart, say out loud a third thing for which you expect to be grateful.

Note: This procedure can be very fast (less than a minute!), and both past and future gratitude items can be one word.

STEP THREE: PAWS2

SECOND PAWS MEASUREMENT (Post-test)

Deep breath. Rate your distress about the original problem from 0 (best) to 10 (worst).

Continue from Step Two until the PAWS number is zero, or the number stays the same for the three measurements.

The Science of the PAWS 🐾 Healing System

- You have physical feelings associated with all of your thoughts. This whole sequence constitutes a pattern interruption. We are working with both positive ideas and positive sensations to interrupt and reshape your neurological patterns around a certain topic.

- Raising eyebrows (surprise response) and smiling (mirth response) both break negative affective patterns, lower stress and trigger euthymia (good feeling) — which is a reason laughter is therapeutic.

- Personality and experimental research demonstrates gratitude is incompatible with bad feeling. You cannot be practicing gratitude and feel anger, fear, or sadness at that time.

- Acupoint tapping research demonstrates stimulating many of these areas causes drops in cortisol, the stress hormone.

- Dropping cortisol disassociates the connection between thoughts of the problem and the stress of having it (breaking classical conditioning). Much of pain, physical or emotional, is the distress the problem causes. Reduce it, and you reduce the pain. Once distress is unpaired from the thought, the connection is broken permanently until relearned.

- The PAWS distress reduction routine blocks right visual field, tied to the left brain, which is the language or "story" part of the brain. It needs to experience change to heal. Blinding the right visual field helps.

- Touching the right side of the face is associated with being comforted as a child.

- Putting a hand over the heart stimulates production of oxytocin (calming and bonding hormone). It also is associated with making a pledge or being deeply touched. Essentially this position is pledging to feel better.

- Combining these effects achieves results that are greater than the sum of the parts.

Spreading the healing yourself

You can teach people to heal too! Tag me on social media (@DrShipon) with the hashtag **#PAWShealer** and I will do my best to post your link on 1MinuteHealing.com. Please also participate in our ongoing research study collecting evidence of efficacy at 1MinuteHealing.com

Here is the script for the demonstration video for you to spread the free healing. It's timed for 60-second Instagram video, several Snapchat snap story segments, etc.

1. "Heal with your paws! Watch me. PAWS stands for Pain, Anger, Worry or Sadness. I'm feeling ____ which I rate as a [0-10] out of 10."

2. Raise eyebrows 3x & smile

3. Perform the PAWS technique.

   a. "Grateful for ___", while right hand over right eye

   b. "Grateful for ___", while right hand on right side of face

   c. "I am already grateful that I will ____" while right hand over your heart

4. "My new PAWS level is a [0-10] out of 10."

5. "You can heal too. Check out 1MinuteHealing.com to learn for free."

My first PAWS healing demonstration video was 45 seconds. I named my wife, my son, and feeling better as my three items. That length seemed right to me.

Foreword

For those of us who've experienced a period of time filled with less than desirable emotions and sensations(which is pretty much all human beings), it can be challenging for the mind to comprehend that one of the most essential ingredients to transforming these experiences is to become enthusiastically grateful for them.

As a formerly stubborn and particularly intellectual psychotherapist in search of constant proof, I required the harsh alarm bell of my apparently dying physical body to open up to seeing the truths outlined in this book.

The chronic pain and chronic illness journey of the medical merry-go-round of doctors, misdiagnoses, treatments, and surgeries left me feeling as if I was a shell of person. I spent years bound to my bed with nowhere to go but within the unexplored areas of my being. I felt forced to get intimately reacquainted with all the monsters I thought I'd dealt with, yet remained hidden inside the shadows of my mind. Any resistance and criticism of them seemed to increase the pain, and by this point, I had enough of that.

So, I tried something new. Something foreign. Something radical: to love the hell out of those misunderstood symptoms and sink deep into gratitude.

Dr. R. Wolf Shipon has written this beautiful guide detailing the very same concept that would mark a turning point in my own transformation. As he states, "Wherever we are warmly received, healing happens." It was during the most traumatic time in my life that I decided to warmly receive myself and every aspect of my current experiences through it all. It's through this unconditional acceptance and appreciation for ourselves and each other that we truly connect with the source of our power and all that fuels each moment: the love of our spirit.

For those who don't fully believe in this concept just yet, I invite you to consider the scientific proof and research outlined in the following pages. While it can feel natural to judge and dismiss what does not appear totally rational, it's only through our willingness to explore the unfamiliar that we actually know the truth.

It's with great pleasure that I hold tremendous gratitude in my heart for the wisdom which Dr. R. Wolf Shipon shares in this book, as well as through all the other platforms we can find him on today.

In love and gratitude,
Jamie Rautenberg, LCSW
Holistic Life & Spiritual Coach
www.thedailyinfusion.com

Introduction

Hi, healer.

I dedicate this to you naturals (autoimmune healers) and you learners (those who seek to become healers based on genuine interest).

If you think you fall into neither category, you probably really fall into the latter because you are reading this. I don't think you are reading this by accident.

This statement about healer "naturals" requires some explanation. I am persuaded by myself and my experiences meeting hundreds of others just like me that everyone who has chronic autoimmune illness or a similar chronic pain condition is in a constant state of seeking a healthy state, with varying degrees of temporary success. This automatically makes them, via their increased sensitivity to pain (in self and others), natural empathic healers.

(The real trick to being and staying empathic is staying upbeat, by the way. You must dose yourself on a huge amount of daily fun, otherwise you become depressed by all the pain you experience and witness. So if you haven't already, lighten up!)

I know this, because writing to you on an overcast day in New Jersey four years after being diagnosed with an autoimmune illness whose needle is somewhere between rheumatoid arthritis, gouty arthritis, and lupus, I struggle almost everyday to feel well. Sometimes I can go long stretches of feeling relatively well, and then it triumphantly returns (these painful homecomings are referred to as flares) which can stretch for days, weeks, even months.

I didn't start my own journey as a healer until almost 20 years ago, doctors thought I had Parkinson's Disease (I had right lateral tremors) and started treating me for it until I learned it was misdiagnosed 18 months later at a Parkinson's clinic. At the time of my misdiagnosis, since nothing any doctor said was making any sense, I went off-script and studied Reiki, a form of Japanese energy medicine. After subsequently teaching Reiki to many others, I learned that I wanted to be a counselor and then a psychologist, but the energy healing journey never ended.

As I wrote in my first book *Reiki Psychology*, this outcome was accurately predicted by one of my Reiki mentors, Nancy Russell of Yardley, PA. "You may think you are a Reiki person who is going to become a psychologist, Wolf," she said. "I would like you to consider the possibility that you are a Reiki person who is going to add psychology to his Reiki practice."

So here I am, nearly 20 years after being made a Reiki master. I run a mid-sized group psychology practice and have a career as a licensed psychologist in which I've written thousands of psychological evaluations and three books. I have been privileged and honored to treat literally hundreds of patients, and I am still yammering on about the very essence of healing based — the energy of gratitude, the topic of my academic research and dissertation.

Today I have learned enough to abbreviate most methods (including Reiki) and save people a lot of time. This happened thanks to extensive training in hypnosis and neurolinguistic programming (NLP), and training/experimentation in the somatic treatments for emotional trauma. And I have learned an incredible lesson about healing in the process: It's all about connection and love.

***

So now for the real kicker. I love you.

Big statement. It's true. I actually love you.

The most interpersonally successful and joyful people in the world almost universally have one amazing quality: they find at least one thing to love (or at least like) about every other person.

It's taken me years — way too long in fact, given both my profession (literally what I *profess* to know and share) and my spiritual inclinations — to arrive here. But if you are reading this, it is literally true and you can test it. And especially if you or someone you love has autoimmune disease, this is something you will grasp faster than others because it's what your system has learned to yearn for: nourishing connection.

Love is not something with which to be stingy. It's not reserved for just a few special people. It's really meant to be for everyone, and the wiser we become the more we understand that the pure universal love of a toddler, kitten or puppy is the most joyful path in the world, and we all strive to return to it.

The more we deploy love, the more powerful it becomes, until it takes on the very quality of healing.

To that end, I offer, if you want yourself or another to heal, you must love. Yourself and everyone else. Unselfishly. Unconditionally. Unerringly.

You will screw up.

You will get angry, hold grudges, and even become avoidant. It's normal. And it's not possible to just love out all the time, every minute you breathe. You will have to set boundaries to protect yourself, your family, your freedom, and even your sanity.

But if you can love everyone, as much as possible, whenever possible, you are absolutely on the path.

The next thing stated here applies whether you are religious or not, secular or of a different religion. Try to extract the reason beyond the religious sentiment, OK? (Try the broccoli, kid!)

My favorite prayer is the Peace Prayer associated with St. Francis of Assisi, which I reproduce here because I say it several times every day and it guides all of me, or at least, I would very much like to think so.

Here it is.

The Peace Prayer of St. Francis of Assisi

Lord, make me an instrument of your peace.
Where there is hatred, let me sow love
Where there is injury, let me sow pardon
Where there is doubt, let me sow faith
Where there is despair, let me sow hope
Where there is darkness, let me sow light
And where there is sadness, let me sow joy.

O Divine Master, grant that I may not so much seek:

To be consoled, as to console
To be understood as to understand
To be loved as to love.

For it is in giving that we receive
It is in pardoning that we are pardoned
And it is in dying to self that we are born to eternal life.
Amen.

I believe this prayer captures the essence of a healer's mission and spirit, but the actual mechanism of healing has its foundation in the emotional practice of gratitude. When gratitude is deployed as a strategy or mechanism, it becomes its most powerful. That is why I am going to teach you, right now in this manual, how to emotionally heal yourself and others.

Chapter 1: The healing power of gratitude

This chapter might be heady, but I need to show you why this stuff works. All the chapters are super short. Stay with me!

The cornerstone of my research for my doctoral degree was shaped into gratitude, after an extensive inventory of my personal beliefs and experiences with regard to mental health and healing. My prior training to Reiki master played no small part in that.

I wanted to author a study showing that <u>gratitude</u>, all by itself, <u>is healing</u>. The process of narrowing down my dissertation to something researchable, that made a valuable contribution to the scientific literature in a reasonable amount of time, changed the nature of what I studied to the effects of gratitude practice on a high-risk group of people with high blood pressure and related problems.

In other words, I needed to get the damned thing done so I had to narrow it down! No joke!

What I found in the process of doing this research, though, was astounding. The connections the study made both inside and outside of its intended topic area were extremely exciting.

In my study, I was able to find statistical support for the notion that people who simply listed five things for which they were deeply in their hearts grateful, every day, had better health outcomes than people who did not do so, even when we controlled for the effects of medication.

Being grateful made things suck less!

In particular, people who practiced gratitude in this way were more likely to:

- Lower their blood pressure
- Lower their measured cynical hostility
- Increase their gratitude levels
- Increase their overall satisfaction with life
- Lose weight
- Quit smoking

This appeared to be support in the direction that I had imagined when I set out to perform my study. I had further support for the notion that the practice of gratitude, by itself, has a healthy component to it.

A great deal of recent scientific work has been done on this by others. The work stretches back to the foundations of some religious beliefs, including Christian Science.

It is not coincidence that gratitude is a component of most religious systems during some of the most important functions (examples include saying grace before meals, and the Mourner's Kaddish in Judaism).

Jews thank God profusely when they mourn. Fascinating, right?

Gratitude is certainly foundational to the practice of Reiki. In fact, in the Reiki Ideals, taught to every beginner in the art, start with two negative injunctions and one remarkable first positive exhortation: "Just for today, do not anger; do not worry and be filled with gratitude."

It appears that many traditions hold gratitude as an essential for mental, emotional, and even spiritual well-being.

In Christian Science, medical doctors are not utilized. Instead, I have been told, adherents to that faith may call a counselor on the phone when ill. The counselor often gets the sick adherent to check his or her "gratitude list" — a list of people who have done something nice for the caller — and make sure that each person on that list has been thanked by the sick adherent for what he or she has done. The process of going through this list, and declaring the gratitude, is for many reasons believed to bring healing to the sick person performing the task, as indicated.

On a related note, in *How to Win Friends and Influence People*, the best-selling business book in the world, gratitude is high-lighted many times by Dale Carnegie as one of the foundational practices to being effective and successful in working with with others.

According to Carnegie, the grateful person has the ability to overcome the greatest social adversity by dint of this disposition. She who starts and ends a request with gratitude is likely to be much more effective in getting that request met, compared to a person who issues a demand — or worse — a complaint.

It's like a criticism sandwich on gratitude bread - begin and end with the good!

Gratitude fits very well into the broaden-and-build theory of positive emotions, as proposed by Dr. Barbara Fredrickson of the University of North Carolina at Chapel Hill. People who practice gratitude have higher levels of creativity, inventiveness, and can see the "big picture" better than those who do not. They are more psychologically resilient, and are more flourishing and expansive in their life paths, than people who do not practice positive emotionality.

The proposed physical healing mechanism

In this book, I propose that research is beginning to offer strong evidence that gratitude practices (feeling-the-feeling of grati-tude then expressing it out loud to self or others) promote positive health states associated with healing and rest.

The physical states are:

- Lowered blood cortisol (the stress hormone)
- Lowered blood pressure
- Increased circulation
- Better diaphragmatic breathing

- Slowed respiration, especially exhalation

In addition, I propose gratitude creates state changes in its recipients and even its witnesses. The state changes that occur to others are:

- Increase in oxytocin release, the bonding hormone

- Increased willingness to deeply listen to the person expressing gratitude

- Increased self-reflection on patterns of prosocial behavior

- Increased likelihood of responding in kind, with their own gratitude, which then cascades into the physical changes described above

- More positive view of others (increased optimism about others and less cynical hostility about people in general)

So all by itself, gratitude is vetted as a healing mechanism. But who can deploy it most effectively, with widest success? I will explain my view on this in the next chapter.

Chapter 2: The healer personality

People of great healing qualities tend to exhibit some of the same personality characteristics and behavior. While this list is certainly not exhaustive, and there are certainly many healers who do not have all these qualities, I have found the cultivation of these five qualities can very well mark a healing personality.

I like to refer to those healers as largely Strifeless, and to me this means that they avoid strife whenever they can.

I conceive of the five characteristics as spelling the phrase: OH GEE!

Here are the five characteristics.

Openness

As defined by the personality researchers behind the personality researchers Paul Costa and Robert McCrae, <u>openness</u> is formally defined as "openness to experience." Here is the definition they have famously used in their research to develop their personality tests:

Openness to Experience: The active seeking and appreciation of experiences for their own sake. This includes the following areas:

1. Fantasy: receptivity to the inner world of imagination
2. Aesthetics: appreciation of art and beauty
3. Feelings: openness to inner feelings and emotions
4. Actions: openness to new experiences on a practical level
5. Ideas: intellectual curiosity
6. Values: readiness to re-examine own values and those of authority figures

Can you see how the healer personality comports with these qualities? Would you feel better around such a person?

Helpfulness

Of course, a healer must have a willingness to help that extends beyond what is normal for others. It must begin with a certain amount of love, and in therapeutic language, we have long used Carl Rogers definition as a starting point.

Unconditional positive regard is known as the basic acceptance and support of a person regardless of what the person says or does.

It reminds me of the definition of *grace* out of the ministry tradition. Grace is defined in Christian belief as the free and unmerited favor of God, as manifested in the salvation of sinners and the bestowal of blessings. In other words, people receive divine help without deserving it. We should be that way, as healers. It doesn't matter who deserves the help. Everyone gets help.

(It reminds me of that episode of Oprah where she declared "Everyone gets a car!" — one of the great moments in talk show history. Check it out on YouTube!)

So everyone gets help, period. Healing is for everyone and so the healer is the best kind of helper. Helpfulness, or even beneficence, is a marked characteristic of the healer personality.

People needs to see this on you. They need to hear it in your voice. They need to feel it in your touch and your hugs. They need to witness it in your behavior. Everything about you should say "This is a helper." Often it means exhibiting the courage to be steadfast even when a person is acting in a vile way, or rejecting you. Stay still, and be helpful when the storm passes.

Gratefulness

The most positive, healing people you know express gratitude on a regular basis. This characteristic can be healing, above all others.

See Chapter 1 for more information about this, but in short:

- Gratitude by itself is foundational to healing practices around the world.

- It is incompatible with bad feelings (especially fear, anger, and sadness).

- When you are in the positive gratitude way of behaving, others feel more comfortable around you.

- In fact, more people want to be around you.

- When you are in a gratitude state, you are likely to be relaxed. People feel more relaxed around relaxed people.

- This leads to the next important point: how that works. All people have mirror neurons in the brain, which replicate behavior witnessed in others. If you are grateful, you create gratitude states in others relying on those mirror neurons that they have. If you can demonstrate gratitude, you can help others have it (they will replicate your behavior, whether they intentionally set out to do that or not), and it will help them heal — and even become healers themselves!

- Finally, gratitude trains the mind to look for the positive. Anything we practice improves over time, including both positive and negative thoughts. The more positively we speak about our lives, the stronger we become at seeing the positive in our own lives and in the lives of others. That is because we are training our neurons to be positive in a positive state. We are reshaping our onboard computers into positive-reason-seeking devices.

These are just some of the many reasons I believe cultivating gratitude states is indoor ant for the healer. "But what if I don't mean it?" I hear you say. "I don't want to be phony!"

You will get over that too, in time. Just practice gratitude. The meaning will occur to you as you do it.

Enthusiasm

Personal experience and more than 20 years in the field of healing and psychology has shown me without a doubt that most the healing people in the world operate from a place of enthusiasm. It's funny, because even in writing this, I had to really struggle between the words "enthusiasm" and "exuberance." While it is true that I like both words very much for teaching this concept, "enthusiasm" is the clear winner.

Think about people you like to be around. How do they treat you? Are they warm to you when they see you, or are they just polite (or worse)?! Are they excited to see you? Would you say that people who seem genuinely thrilled to see you are some of your favorite people to be around, spend time with, or work with on any given day?

If your answers were yes, you're like most people. If your answers were no, you are weird.

No, I don't really mean that, but there might be some differences in the way you developed your preferences that are going to make this concept a little harder to understand, so sit tight and I'll explain it. Hang in there. I'm going to confirm the biases of other people and try to change yours! I write that with love and respect (and a little grin).

Warmly being received heals a person all by itself. You can be warmly received and therefore healed a little in many places, not just necessarily with someone who really performs a healing art. I live in New Jersey, where there are lots of restaurants known as diners. Being warmly received by the staff changes the whole experience, and the best family diners know that. People are warmly received at their local watering holes (remember the show "Cheers" and the opening number? "Sometimes you wanna go where everybody knows your name / and they're always glad you came / you wanna be where you can see our troubles are all the same / you wanna be where everybody knows your name"). People are warmly received at churches, synagogues, and mosques. People are warmly received on the golf course, the hairdresser, and even at the delicatessen. Wherever they are warmly received, healing happens.

I literally make it my business to be warm in my reception of others, and it works. I learned one lesson in this from my wife. She suggested I offer tea and even a snack to everyone who comes in to talk at our psychology practice, and it makes us stand out. Do you know I have peers who are so cheap they want to charge the client the credit card transaction fee, let alone even think about giving them tea or a snack? Come on. That's not warm, and it's certainly not enthusiastic! That kind of behavior seldom works to make people feel welcomed.

Enthusiasm means so much more than being welcoming, however. We can be warm and welcoming me and still not enthusiastic in our approach to things, or other people.

When I see you, I want to be *excited* about even the *chance* to see you. When I talk to you, I want to be fully *interested and engaged* in whatever you're talking about, and if I'm honestly not, I've learned that it is not the fault of the other person. I learned that from a very wise lady named Dr. Marjorie Levitt, a professor of psychology and a gestalt therapist. She taught our class of nine doctoral students that "boredom is the active decision to withhold interest from others" — which means if we are bored, it is incumbent upon us to discover what part of us deciding to withhold interest from the other person (and resolve it).

Our natural state is fascination and wonder, which is what we all had in early childhood. If that is not happening, it is morally incumbent upon us to analyze why and use that information to find a way to reconnect.

Being filled with interest, warmth and excitement about the other person is the foundation of this thing I am calling enthusiasm, and now for the kicker: the word itself describes its own power. You have to dig into how the word came to be to unlock it.

Enthusiasm comes from the Greek word *enthousiasmos,* from *enthousiazein,* which means "to be inspired" — and — wait for it — *entheos,* inspired, from *en theos,* which is "In God" or "In the Divine."

Enthusiasm is being filled with the presence of inspiration, the presence of spirit, the divine. It's being that present, the tuned in, that excited. And if you're not an inspired person, if you want to be a healer, it is your responsibility to get that in your life however you need to get it. Some people get it from music. Some get it from contact with nature, ministry and affirmation healing (such as the ministries of Joel Osteen or the healing messages of Louise Hay), inspirational speakers like Tony Robbins, business leaders like Gary Vaynerchuk and Seth Godin, experimenters like Tim Ferriss, good news stories, socializing, dancing, having deep conversations in person or with new people on social media (such as on my favorite platform for it: www.Anchor.fm).

However you need to get it, go get it and dose yourself on different kinds of inspiration regularly, and see how it changes your enthusiasm as defined here.

I heard an expression once: "People don't care about how much you know until they know how much you care." If you are not in the enthusiastic place in making contact with others, healing is going to be very hard. Get inspired. It's infectious, and just like with gratitude, if you are enthusiastic, you will create it in the people around you. You will create healers where you once only brought healing.

Expectancy

While all of the others stand tall as great characteristics of people who heal, this last one towers above them all as the most important feature against depression and in favor of optimism.

Hold onto your hats, everyone. This is the most difficult personality characteristic to cultivate!

Expectancy, or specifically positive expectancy, distinguishes itself as the faith that all circumstances will work out for the good, or at least that a healing sense of peace is possible, even when things look really bad. It is the essence of optimism, and to me it requires a person to have great trust in the universe or the divine influence if it is based in circumstance; if the positive expectancy rejects circumstance, it is based in knowledge of how healing peace is possible no matter what happens in the world.

Allow me to explain, because this gets deep. It comes down to basic worldview, and before we discuss this fully, it might be helpful to talk about at what level the thinking has to occur. For expectancy, it should be at the deepest level, so let's discuss the levels.

In cognitive therapy, there are two levels of thought: automatic thoughts and core beliefs.

An *automatic thought* is something that we think immediately in response to a set of circumstances. So for instance, an automatic thought when someone cuts you off on the highway might be "What a jerk!" If a person is seeking cognitive therapy for anger or even depression, a cognitive therapist might look at that automatic thought and say to the client, "Can you think of any other possible thoughts to have under the circumstance of getting cut off on the highway?" This would be a challenging question for many people, but ultimately that person may come up with, "Well, the driver could have been having an emergency" or "He could have been avoiding something in the road" or "Maybe I was in his blind spot and he didn't see me."

Much of the early stages of therapy, in this model, is helping people come up with alternative thoughts that are less extreme than the automatic thoughts already being used. By making the thoughts more "scientific" and open to possibilities, the emotions and resulting behaviors become less extreme as well, and the person begins to feel better.

A *core belief* lives within a person as a basic assumption about the world. Often these are limited to a small handful, and constitutes kind of a template for all of life. It is the ultimate source of most of those automatic thoughts, and it usually reveals itself after several sessions of cognitive therapy. Often it is the therapist who pieces it together while working with the person, and it's usually a fairly basic idea. That same driver who had the automatic thought "What a jerk!" when she was cut off may have the basic core belief such as "People cannot be trusted" or "No one cares (about me or anyone else)." Do you see how this basic core belief as a template would color nearly everything about the world? Core beliefs exist at a very deep level, and are very slow to change, if they can be changed at all. They respond very slowly to contrary evidence presented on a very regular basis. One can dose oneself on this contrary evidence, but the danger in doing it alone is our own confirmation bias. We usually seek out information that confirms our core beliefs (which is why politically polarized media outlets do so well).

Now for the heavy part! The healer must have a core belief that all is well, and all will be well in the future.

The most healing characteristic a person can have is *hope*, the essence of positive expectancy. But it is not a weak hope, like "Oh, I hope that works out." It is a powerful hope, an unshakable belief that all must work out. It is a conviction. Anthony Robbins says that people will live or die by their convictions, and this is an incredibly important sensibility to have about hope.

There is going to be a difference in the core beliefs of Western believers and Eastern-thinking healers about healing outcomes, so let's make the distinction and move on. A Western believer is going to believe something like "God has a plan, He can directly intervene in this set of circumstances, and even if it doesn't work out the way I was hoping, God has a better plan even if we don't understand it." By contrast, positive expectancy in the Eastern tradition might be more like "Peace and spiritual healing are always possible in any physical circumstance, and my goal is to work toward the highest possible good which is rooted in warmth, non-struggle, and ultimately acceptance."

There are some people who are able to combine these beliefs in a way that makes sense to them, or whose beliefs are so flexible that they can take parts of one and apply it to the other. Most people may have difficulty with that, but I thought it was important to point out that both of these beliefs are their own forms of positive expectancy and can be found in many healers.

Now, this is important. Decide where you stand. Meditate, pray, or both. Go inside and find out what your positive expectancy is about the future, and what its spiritual or philosophical basis is, and then you can proceed by getting it rooted deep down using the following method to become the healer you really want to be.

Chapter 3: The Healer Initiation

Remember the cheat sheet in the beginning of this manual?

I am going to replicate it here, and not just because I want you to know my face! I am doing it because becoming a healer can be a daily or even hourly decision, and just like anything else you practice, it gets stronger over time.

The beautiful thing about this method is that the very self-same practices you would use to deeply heal another person are the ones would use on yourself to calibrate your system to heal others, whether your are using the PAWS method with them, or are just in their presence to heal them. Here is how you do it.

STEP ONE:

FIRST HEALING INFLUENCE MEASUREMENT (HIM Pre-test)

Rate your own sense of being filled with healing power from 0 (best) to 10 (worst).

Raise your eyebrows 3 times, then smile (even forced — fake it until you make it)!

Deep breath in, and slow exhale.

STEP TWO:

Do the PAWS positions!

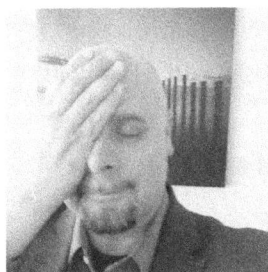

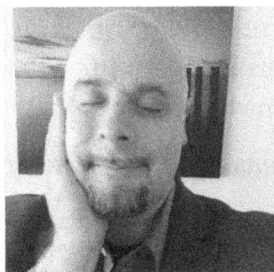

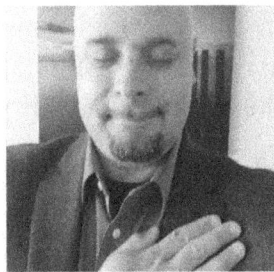

Note: Eyes may be open or closed. This guy likes his eyes closed.

1. Right palm over right eye, mitten-like fingers of right hand (held together) on forehead, say outloud one way you are Open-Helpful-Grateful-Enthusiastic-Expectant (OH GEE)

2. Mitten-like right hand on right side of face, say outloud a second OH GEE

3. Mitten-like hand over heart, say outloud a third OH GEE

Note: This procedure can be very fast (less than a minute!). Do the OH GEEs in sequence, whether you're doing 5 sequences with 3 of each (recommended for beginners) or doing a "quickie" (one Openness, one Helpfulness, one Gratitude, one Enthusiastic, and one Expectant, and finish again with Gratitude for the sixth position).

STEP THREE:

SECOND HIM MEASUREMENT (Post-test)

Deep breath. Rate your own sense of being filled with healing power from 0 (best) to 10 (worst).

Continue from Step Two until the HIM number is at a level you are satisfied, or the number stays the same for the three measurements.

How it works

So just like with the PAWS method, you are relying on using physical and ideational stimuli to reshape your patterns about being a healer.

In this method, you are relying on your own personal story about the OH GEE patterns in your life to inculcate or strengthen the healing sensibility in your life.

So, with respect to increasing your capacity as a healer:

- You have physical feelings associated with all of your thoughts. This whole sequence constitutes a pattern interruption. We are working with both positive ideas and positive sensations to interrupt and reshape your neurological patterns around a certain topic, in this case, *being a healer.*

- Raising eyebrows (surprise response) and smiling (mirth response) both break negative affective patterns, lower stress and trigger euthymia (good feeling) — which is a reason laughter is therapeutic. *Your ability to laugh is part of being a healer.*

- All of these states (Openness, Helpfulness, Gratefulness, Enthusiasm, and Expectancy) are being translated from merely ideas into physical states by this practice. You are using the power of neurolinguistic programming (NLP) to repattern ideational data into physical sensation, and then rehearsing it.

- Acupoint tapping research demonstrates stimulating many of these areas causes drops in cortisol, the stress hormone. *The lower your stress, the better you heal.*

- *As cortisol drops your healing attention increases.* When you have lower cortisol levels, you can use more of your prefrontal cortex to focus your attention on the other person, which is what the person receiving healing so deeply craves.

- Touching the right side of the face is associated with being comforted as a child. *You need to have that comforted-and-comforting sensibility in order to heal.*

- Putting a hand over the heart stimulates production of oxytocin (calming and bonding hormone). *Your ability to bond is healing too, and people pick up on this.*

- Combining these effects achieves results that are greater than the sum of the parts.

As your feelings about being a healer change, so do your behaviors. Everything you feel comes across in your physicality and is telegraphed to the people around you. This is a most important realization when it comes to *being a healer. How you feel is what the other person will feel.*

I strongly suggest making time once per day to do the healer initiation. If you don't have time to perform the full version, just do the two passes with OH GEE-G.

Buddhism teaches that what compassion we have for ourselves is the compassion we have for others, and vice versa. We know that what we witness others performing physically affects the same areas of our brains as if we were physically doing the same things.

In other words, we are all deeply connected. If you really want to heal others, you must be deeply healed. I believe that the deepest form of healing the world is healing the self, and the deepest form of healing the self is healing the world. Whatever you can do to brighten your world brightens you inside, and whatever brightens you inside brightens the world.

Go brighten, both ways.

Chapter 4: Healing others

We spent the last chapter talking about becoming a healer. In this chapter, I am going to talk with you about how to use the PAWS method to heal others, and also how to directly use your own hands to heal another person who is in very close, personal relationship to you.

Teaching others the PAWS method

One of the greatest gifts you can give another person is teaching them how to feel better. While, naturally, I would like people to know about this manual and watch any videos about the method online, *no one can replace a personal connection with a book or a video.*

That is why I see anyone teaching this method as a healer. Sitting with someone and walking them through the method, just as you learned it here and maybe through a video, is so much more meaningful than directing them to a video. It helps the person heal better when there is a personal connection.

So here's what you do.

1. A healing interaction begins by creating a non-distracted place to fully hear the problem, and to listen as much with your eyes and heart as your ears. Get into privacy, preferably in person.

2. Hear the problem and identify the accompanying feeling (not the thought). As a basic rule, Paul Ekman defined the six basic universal emotions. He later identified many more. Here are the basic six followed by the more recent additions. First, identify the feeling. Negative ones that you are likely to be working with are bolded for clarity.

a. **Anger**
b. **Disgust**
c. **Fear**
d. Happiness
e. **Sadness**
f. Surprise
g. Amusement
h. **Contempt**
i. Contentment
j. **Embarrassment**
k. Excitement
l. **Guilt**
m. Pride in achievement
n. Relief
o. Satisfaction
p. Sensory pleasure
q. **Shame**

3. Have the person rate the distress created by the negative feeling (a, b, c, e, h, j, l, or q above) from 0-10, 10 being the worst (broad categories, if you want to use them instead, are Pain Anger Worry or Sadness, or PAWS levels).

4. Talk them through the whole PAWS method (don't forget to have them raise their eyebrows three times in the beginning, and smile!) using present or past **gratitude** (first 2 positions) or anticipated **future gratitude** (last position).

5. Get that PAWS level as close to zero as you can. Stop when at zero or when the number stays the same for three PAWS post-tests.

6. Give them a copy of the cheat sheet in the front of this manual so they can practice. There are also directions on PAWShealer.com and 1MinuteHealing.com

Utilizing 3-Point Healing Touch

If you've practiced initiating yourself as described in this section, on a regular basis, and/or if you are trained in other hands-on healing modalities, you can use a variant of the PAWS method on others. I call it 3-Point Healing Touch.

This is important: Unless you have a legal license to touch (you are a medical doctor, nurse, medical assistant, massage therapist, acupuncturist, reflexologist, chiropractor, etc), do not use the person-to-person physical parts of this method with others unless you are very close to them (family member, romantic partner, or very close friend you have known a long time). This method will not serve others well if you become their healer physically. Your greatest gift is teaching people how to heal themselves, and you can do that by teaching them the simple PAWS method.

With that out of the way, here is how you can do it.

1. As above, have them describe the problem and how it makes them feel (refer to Ekman's list, above). Have them rate the PAWS level of that negative feeling from 0-10, 10 being the worst.

2. Ask if you may put your hands on the person to help that person feel better.

3. You can skip the eyebrow and smiling part. This whole interaction represents so much of a pattern interruption that it is not necessary in this set of circumstances.

4. Place your right hand on the person's left shoulder and your left hand (fingers together as mittens and thumb with fingers) on the person's forehead, and have that person name one thing for which he is grateful.

5. Move your left hand to the person's right side of the face, fingers together as a mitten, and have that person name another thing for which he is grateful.

6. Move your left hand to the person's right shoulder, land have that person name something for which he is <u>hopeful</u>.

7. Have them do their PAWS level. Repeat until the number gets to 0 or is consistent for three tries.

8. Give the other person a hug! If it's someone really close, make it up to 20 seconds for the maximum oxytocin release.

9. Tell them about the PAWS method available on 1MinuteHealing.com or PAWShealer.com so they can learn and spread the word. Invite them to participate in our research study too!

This acts as a powerful form of healing for people who are close to you. It causes the release of oxytocin in others, the same as getting a massage or a hug, but the cognitive exercise of using gratitude and expectancy works to change people faster than just being comforted.

I am partial to people healing themselves. I always have been, but some people need someone to intervene for them.

This is very important: If you are working with someone professionally without a license to touch, avoid being drawn into the touch-healing role. Save it for family members, romantic interests, and other loved ones.

The pattern interruption of the basic PAWS method is much more powerful because it is more portable, you can use it anywhere, and you don't need another person to do it for you.

Teach a person to fish.

Teach a person to heal.

Chapter 5: The Wounded Healers

I operate from the supposition that people with chronic illness of any kind (mental/physical) are more intimately aware of suffering than others. It is because it this that I propose that they make the most qualified healers. For them, healing is not merely academic or a trade. It is a necessity for living, and it needs to happen daily in order to survive.

Because I struggle with chronic pain (autoimmune illness - a nonspecific inflammatory illness like Lupus and RA which affects every joint in my body) as well as the often accompanying depression (which had been in remission for several years, thank God), I am more sensitive to these things than many others. I believe this gives me a huge advantage in treating other people with chronic pain and depression.

But I am not terribly unique. I believe there are so many people, and maybe you yourself, who can and will be better healers than I can be in many ways.

A known phenomenon

The wounded healer is a well known human archetype.

From Wikipedia, our modern day hive-mind (thanks, Star Trek):

Wounded healer is a term created by psychologist Carl Jung. The idea states that an analyst is compelled to treat patients because the analyst himself is "wounded". The idea may have Greek mythology origins. Research has shown that 73.9% of counselors and psychotherapists have experienced one or more wounding experiences leading to their career choice.

This idea has its origins even in Greek mythology. The great centaur Chiron was a healer and teacher wounded by an arrow of Hercules. Jung himself admitted to being a wounded healer.

Certainly, his mentor Sigmund Freud, whose entire theoretical system was based on a self-analysis, could be named one. And today, there are so many examples in popular cultures, including the protagonists of *House* and *Nurse Jackie.*

Jung would have said that with this story as an archetype, or one of the great stories common to our consciousness as members of the human race, there is something special about our relationship to it. The truth is that wounded healers are throughout the healing professions and traditions, from traditional to nontraditional. Some of the fields in which I have witnessed wounded healers in abundance include the following: internal medicine, physiatry, psychiatry, chiropractic, naturopath doctors, homeopathy, traditional psychology/counseling/social work, special education, physical education, physical therapy, occupational therapy, music therapy, addictions counseling, clinical hypnosis, Christian ministry, Buddhist teaching, Ayurvedic medicine and yoga, meditation, shamanic healing, energy work of all kinds (including Reiki, Qigong, Healing Touch, Integrative Energy Therapy etc), psychics, mediums, tarot readers, crystal healers and herbalists and nutritionists of various stripes and pedigrees.

Did you find yourself surprised seeing some of those practices listed together in the same sentence? Some people might even be offended! The truth is we all have many things in common. Among them: contextualizing human suffering into a system of understanding, and seeking to alleviate it.

In other words, every one of those practices has its foundation in seeking to help. In compassion. In love.

The Autoimmune Healer

I believe so many people are like me, with their own immune systems attacking healthy tissue, there has to be an evolutionary purpose. I choose to believe, with no evidence to support this by the way, that people with autoimmune illness all have the experience of contrast in abundance. Most experience times when they feel relatively well, and then times they feel much worse (flares) — sometimes lasting for part of a day, and sometimes for months!

Because we have this experience of contrast, we are familiar with highs and lows, ease and disease, pleasure and pain, weakness and strength, all on an unpredictable time table. The good days are so much better by having the bad days.

I choose to believe that people with autoimmune disease, therefore, have a calling to healing. There is no known cure for these conditions. So, it would make sense that a class of people with chronic illness, who are always seeking ways to feel better themselves, would become content experts and distributors of information when it comes to feeling better. In other words, they are well positioned experientially to be healers and teachers.

So what if we call people with autoimmune disease, and others who have chronic conditions, naturals? People who understand healing so intimately, because they yearn for it for so much of their daily lives?

We are all healers

As life goes on, the challenges with which we are faced tend to increase in number. Age can beget physical problems at some point, relationships and circumstances change, and the temporary nature of all things requires a higher perspective in order to negotiate with any sense of peace or enduring wholeness.

As these processes occur, we have to make meaning out of it. Perhaps the struggles we face serve us to help others suffer less. Maybe, in some ways, we learn best by contrast. Having difficult times makes the good times so much sweeter.

Making sense of it presents us with an enormous challenge. Contextualizing sadness, fear, pain, and loss into a joyful overall life experience requires a healer, and no matter who you are, the greatest healer you lives within yourself.

We are all healers, so keep healing.

Chapter 6: Hush the Narrator (Meditation)

Note: I believe the 1MinuteHealing.com system is complete and effective. I am including other healing systems I use in my practice in these sections of the book in order to offer an expanded under-standing of the concepts that have been woven into the PAWS system.

If you are reading this guide, it is likely you are a healer.

It is also likely that you have a first-person narrator in your head.

As far as I know, we all do. I have one too. My inner narrator is usually saying things like:

"What is there for me to eat?"
"How much longer is this going to take?"
"What is the next thing I have to do right now?"
"I kind of hope that person doesn't talk to me." (In the elevator)
"Can't I get around this guy?" (In traffic)

But sometimes my internal narrator also says things like:
"If I don't complete this today, I'll never get it done/fail/etc."
"That person doesn't seem to like me too much."
"How am I going to pay the bills if...?"

And when things get really bad, the narrator says things like:
"I'm no good at that."
"I have no business trying to be friends with that person."
"I'm   a   lousy son/husband/friend/businessperson/coworker/etc."
"I'm so sad/angry/anxious/tense I can't stand it."
"If I don't [fill in the blank] I'm going to lose it."

So, I'm just like you. I am not enlightened about very many things (though I know a few things about healing), I certainly have not reached Nirvana (sounds kind of boring, to be honest), and have no special claim to total tranquility or impervious mental health. In fact, I became a healer because I need to heal.

But here's the thing: The voice talking about my life in my head isn't me. And your internal narrator isn't you talking either.

Both ancient and modern mindfulness meditation practice is about noticing thoughts, and recognizing that the thoughts are not us. They are just thoughts.

René Descartes is famous for stating (in French), "I think, therefore I am." Most Western thought-about-thought agrees with that: We are what we think (kind of like: "You are what you eat").

But what if it's not true?

Change the story

Well, for one thing, it would mean that the story we tell ourselves all day is just a story. And thus, the "story of ourselves" which is constantly replaying for us in our heads may be subject to revision.

What if we could revise our stories so that they were more positive, forthright, creative, permissive, forgiving, and less stressed-out?

Could this enhance us as healers?

As a psychologist, I know of several tools for becoming more positive. One is psychotherapy itself. Psychotherapy is a tried-and-true tool to get a person to examine his or her own thoughts and behaviors, and modify them to feel better and do better in life. The psychotherapist has the unique role of highlighting any of the client's thoughts that may not work so well so that the client can change them. A good therapist also highlights what has worked well, so the client can keep thinking that way.

People write in diaries and journals sometimes for this self-examination (and often review entries with a psychotherapist). And people read many self-help books, watch inspirational speakers, look to holy books for guidance, and seek advice from friends and family to change their thoughts all the time. We even have a colloquialism for this (and we know from neurolinguistic programming that colloquialisms carry the wisdom of the culture): "I changed my mind." You can change your mind anytime you want.

Why changing the story in your mind is hard

The reason people do not change their minds, and their stories, all the time, is because they have not accepted the premise that every thought they have is likely to be fictional.

There is no such thing as a thought that totally captures the truth (all thoughts merely symbolize reality, and so these symbols, by definition, cannot define the nuanced essence of anything).

This is one of the underpinnings of a set of consulting and communication techniques called neurolinguistic programming (NLP): Every thought is either a useful or non-useful *fiction*. In NLP, you are encouraged to select the *useful fictions* over the non-useful fictions.

So most of us, most of the time, have a bunch of thoughts narrating our experience and we assume those thoughts are "true." By doing so, we are at a double disadvantage: There is no such thing as true, and we don't have anyone to help dispute our secret thoughts for us.

That is why meditation is so helpful. Mindfulness meditation exercises the power of the person to look at those secret thoughts dispassionately, and let them go. The mental calisthenics of seeing a thought as just a thought and then letting it go allows you to do this in future situations that may really bother you. But you probably cannot perform the letting it go act efficiently or well without having repeatedly and habitually done the mental calisthenics of this kind of meditation.

If you are like me, there are minor to major annoyances often in your daily experience. That is why I have to recommend to you meditation: to improve your mind. We want to build a better brain, and we should create one that handles stress better than it does now. This will allow you to more quickly quiet the noise of your inner narrator, and move on to experiencing your world in a more meaningful way, with higher reserves of mental energy.

This can only enhance your practice as a healer.

The World's Shortest Guide to Mindfulness Meditation

There is so much guidance in the world on mindfulness meditation, that all you really need is a short how-to. If you want more details, gosh, there are plenty of them available on Google/YouTube.

1. Find a place to sit comfortably for at least five minutes, and set at least a 5 minute timer (I use an iPhone app called "Insight Timer" which has cool social media features).

2. Sit up straight, close your eyes or keep them half-closed, and breathe.

3. Focus on the sensation of breathing in and out. You may feel breath near your nose, your mouth, your chest, or your abdomen.

4. Your mind will wander. That's the whole point. As you lose your focus on the breath and notice your mind wandering to something else, just acknowledge that it wandered (i.e. Say to yourself: "Hmm") and then focus on your breathing again until your mind wanders again.

5. Don't feel bad about your mind wandering. In fact, feel good about it. It's actually the whole "point of the game" (in fact, I see it as a built-in video game of sorts). You will bring your thoughts back to your breath, for as long as you can, until it wanders again.

6. Alternative technique tip for a quick fix: Try breathing in compassion for yourself, breathe out a longer breath of compassion for others. This is a meditation that is being used to avoid "compassion fatigue" among caregivers. It also helped me get my baby to sleep. Another tip might be to envision a flower opening on inhalation, closing on exhalation, and keeping your focus on that.

Sound boring? Well, what is boredom? Is that the narrator talking (like mine just did about Nirvana)? Hey, do as I say, not as I do!

Once you complete your five minutes, two things will have happened:

- You will be in the new habit of noticing that thoughts are just thoughts, and not "you."

- You will be able to carry out dismissals of bothersome thoughts more easily in your daily life.

This is the first step in a liberation from the tyrannical narrator that we assume is "ourselves" when in fact, the narration is just a series of thoughts that do not have to define any of us, and especially not you.

By beginning with mindfulness meditation, you are liberating your brain and reclaiming it to work for your own purposes (Healing! Remember?), and not some kind of automatic (mindless) purpose that will drive you to distraction and unhappiness.

Your most upsetting thought is not what is really happening. It is merely a thought.

Just a story told by your narrator.

Chapter 7: Expanded Healing (Compassion)

Note: I believe the PAWS system is complete and effective. I am including other healing systems I use in my practice in these sections of the book in order to offer an expanded understanding of the concepts that have been woven into the PAWS system.

Healing is based in compassion. Compassion has its foundation in love.

Many practitioners of Buddhism often sit in their meditations and reflect on sending love and compassion to all the creatures on Earth. They especially focus on sending those feelings to people who may have wronged them or behaved very badly toward other people. This is called Metta, or the Compassion Meditation.

The benefits of being nicer inside

Research is beginning to indicate that the Compassion Meditation is very good for people. Studies have indicated that it increases feelings of social connectedness, reduces pain and anger in people with chronic lower back pain, and boosts positive emotions and feelings of well-being in life. It may even lower inflammation and even change the way the emotional part of the brain works. That is pretty neat for a practice that simply focuses on sending loving kindness to others, and then sending it back the self. Maybe "All You Need Is Love," after all.

Various techniques developed over the past 2,500 years

I have learned about several different forms of Metta, and some of them take longer than others. The traditional Metta exercise recognizes that life features suffering (the First Noble Truth of Buddhism) and that, despite that, all creatures desire to be happy. This is the exercise I use with my therapy clients and those who consult with me. It is healing all by itself. Though not as fast or flashy as PAWS, it has incredible merit for a healer. Especially a *world healer.*

How it may save the world

So let us just follow some far-out logic for a minute. Human beings are the greatest risk to the planet, and also the only species with the capacity for saving it from, say, a planet-killing asteroid. The human species — with the potential to be the "guardian species" of the planet — is still evolving all the time. In fact, we can consume foods (simple carbohydrates) that could not be consumed by humans 5,000 years ago. If children you know are playing video games you cannot comprehend, it could be because the visual cortex may be evolving between generations, as some evidence seems to suggest.

The great evidence for human superiority is the human brain, and it can be used for very selfish, petty, and unenlightened purposes. But the human has the capacity to evolve his own brain faster than any other species, by getting the brain to work on itself (through a process known as metacognition, or thinking-about-thinking).

Metacognition is performed by reflection, education, practice, discipline, and disciplined meditation. As the human brain evolves with compassion for other humans and all living creatures, the world changes because — at least to our current knowledge — it is the human brain that has the greatest impact on the planet as a whole.

Did you fully appreciate that? At least as far as we know, only humans have the capacity to destroy or heal Planet Earth.

Finally, since quantum physics and ancient spiritualities both teach in various ways that separation between objects, distance, and time are all illusions based on our location within the space-time continuum, then everything is really intimately connected to everything else. What you think about becomes part of the Whole, because nothing is separated from anything else.

So maybe "Everything is Really One Thing."

Maybe I am you, and you are me, and all of we are connected to everything else, and...

If so, by meditating on compassion, you/we get a votes in the cosmic order as part of our conscious connection to All That Is. Your mind is a broadcaster. You can air good programs. Assume the broadcast will be received by the greater audience, and will influence that audience.

Pretty heavy when you consider that in the context of healing, right?

Along those lines, we can perhaps believe that for at least the past 2,500 years, the people who have been praying and meditating for good things have been having some say in how things unfolded. For instance, the human race has not annihilated itself and all other life yet, though we have had the capacity to do exactly that for the past 70 years. Maybe the compassion meditation and prayer has had an impact, after all.

The human race will evolve to the point that it will minimize the amount of suffering it causes the other species of the Earth, but it will take time. You can accelerate the process by practicing kindness to others, kindness to yourself, and kindness to all creatures — and teaching others to do the same. This may be the greatest thing that we can learn, and it is here (and many other places) in a few short pages. It must begin in the mind, and it must be a daily and serious — while still joyful — undertaking.

It begins with you, healer.

The World's Shortest Guide to Compassion Meditation (Metta)

Think of at least five people, in order, from the nearest and dearest person to you, to a person with whom you disagree or whose behavior you find highly objectionable (someone doing horrible things).

You will say the following script to each person, taking time to think of his or her suffering and wishing to alleviate it.

The Script

"May you be happy. May you be healthy. May you be safe. May you live with ease."

This is just one variant. Sometimes I have heard, "May you be free of pain and suffering. May you be happy and live in peace." I have also heard, "May you be free of suffering. I care about your suffering. May your life be happy. I love you."

You get to pick the words that work for you.

Then you will say The Script back to yourself, wishing yourself the same. The key is this: Your script must be the same for everyone. Say it even if you don't mean it. Everyone gets the same treatment, or as Oprah said, "Everyone gets a car! You get a car! And you get a car!"

You really have to watch that old Oprah clip.

The Process

1. Think of someone dearest to you, and recite The Script. Then say The Script, wishing it to yourself.

2. Think of the next closest person, and recite The Script. Then wish it to yourself.

3. Think of the third closest person (neutral), and recite The Script. Then wish it to yourself.

4. Think of the fourth person (a little difficult), and recite The Script. Then wish it to yourself.

5. Think of the fifth person (the most difficult), and recite The Script. Then wish it to yourself.

6. As a bonus (and I think this is the best part) envision taking a mental and spiritual road trip around the world, seeing all the people and all the creatures of the land, sea, and air. Wish them all The Script. Then wish it to yourself.

What's the point?

Your Compassion meditation practice exists for you. While I do hope that it has an impact on the wider world (the broadcasting bit I referenced above), this is chiefly a tool for your own well-being from a strictly positive-life-change point of view.

If you view the mind as a muscle, compassion for yourself is a skill. There is no difference between the nerves that handle compassion for yourself and the nerves that handle it for the other people as represented in your brain.

We all have the capacity for cruelty and callousness, as well as love and caring. Aside from caring being an evolutionary goal, the fields of cognitive and positive psychology are revealing that people who have consistently kind thoughts of themselves, others, and the future are happier and better adjusted than those who are hostile and cynical.

When you state your compassion for the person nearest to you, and turn it toward yourself, you benefit from that warm level of feeling. When you state it for a neutral person, and turn it toward yourself, you benefit from the natural level of feeling you are willing to extend to a neutral person. And quite importantly, when you extend compassion to a person whose actions you strongly dislike, you accomplish a mental and emotional feat that stretches your morality and kindness. Extending compassion to yourself after accomplishing that is very rewarding and shows you what a big person you can be.

Oh, and it's healing.

There is something to be said for the cognitive capacity to convince ourselves we are good. We do not get a lot of practice at that, and we need to practice it to undo the years of self-critical thought that creeps in over time. The self-critical thought limits us more than we know.

Finally, it will be easier for you to be nice to others. Your resulting wellbeing can be read in your micro-expressions how you feel, and people will treat you according to what they consciously or unconsciously perceive as the improvements in your expressions, postures, and tones of voice.

While it is tempting to say that Compassion is the most important part of this healing system, that would be unfair because Mindfulness is a true process of standing apart from thought, and Gratitude is a very effective tool for overall wellbeing as exemplified in the PAWS system.

In other words, as my favorite hippies have always said, "It's all good!" But compassion, yes. Love. Love is where it is all at.

Chapter 8: Self-Soothing Hands (SSH)

Note: I believe the 1MinuteHealing.com system is complete and effective. I am including other healing systems I use in my practice in these sections of the book in order to offer an expanded understanding of the concepts that have been woven into the PAWS system.

Touch comforts.

When you stub your toe, you reach down to touch it. When you have a toothache, you touch the side of your face. When you have a headache, you touch your head.

When a child falls down, you kiss the boo-boo to make it better. When another person hurts inside, you are probably inclined to give that person a hug.

If you are friends with an animal such as a dog or a cat, you may notice that when you are physically hurting or in emotional pain/exhaustion, the animal spends time very near to you.

A new way to think about healing

There is a reason for all of this. Practitioners of Reiki and similar touch-healing modalities explain that there is an energy, or life-force, that is shared among all living beings. When we are hurt, the impulse to touch is the impulse to comfort. The comfort may not occur from the mere application of pressure or heat from touching, but rather, from some other aspect of it. In Reiki, it is thought that the universal life-force energy (from whence the term rei-ki is derived) is what is being transmitted in that moment. According to the tradition, a universal, benign, nondenominational, soothing and healing energy, is available to all creatures to utilize when they hurt. Fascinating idea.

Foundations of gratitude for feeling better

Before I became a counselor, and then a psychologist, I was hurting badly due to some physical problems which made no sense medically, and so I learned Reiki. Then I started teaching it to others.

I encountered a fascinating idea from a grad school professor I had at the time. She was a Christian Scientist. She said that when people in her church get sick, instead of using doctors, they call a gratitude counselor on the telephone. The gratitude counselor has the sick person review his or her "gratitude list" — quite literally a list of people whom the sick person owed a "thank you." Once this list was reviewed, the sick person's job was to go thank the people who had helped. This was supposed to resolve illness. (The theological underpinning of the practice is also interesting. Christian Science founder Mary Baker Eddy believed that gratitude for eternal life is what raised Lazarus from the dead.)

What I discovered is that the practice of gratitude, internally, was already part of Reiki practice. Mrs. Hawayo Takata, who taught Reiki to the West, transmitted these principles for practicing Reiki:

The Reiki Ideals

> *The secret art of inviting happiness*
> *The miraculous medicine of all diseases*
> *Just for today, do not anger*
> *Do not worry and be filled with gratitude*
> *Devote yourself to your work. Be kind to people*
> *Every morning and evening, join your hands in prayer*
> *Pray these words to your heart*
> *and chant these words with your mouth*
> *Usui Reiki Treatment for the improvement of body and mind*
>   *— The founder, Mikao Usui*

A modified traditional Reiki practice

Since the first positive instruction of the Reiki Ideals, as related above, was to "be filled with gratitude" (as opposed to all of the things you should avoid, like angering and worrying), it made sense to me that gratitude is the foundational feeling of Reiki. This led me to my research, which was to determine whether gratitude is a good foundational feeling state for health in general.

When I was teaching Reiki to dozens of students, I learned that gratitude is what helped people "warm up their hands" faster than any of my other instructions. So I took a shortcut. Gratitude is a foundational idea to healing, so it would serve as a quick way to teach Reiki.

What I am teaching you here cannot be considered traditional Reiki teaching. It can, however, be considered a shortcut approach to activating an internal state that may be the same, near, or even superior to the state you may experience if you were traditionally taught Reiki.

This is one of the tools I teach because it provides a soothing and relaxation modality that is different from most other therapies.

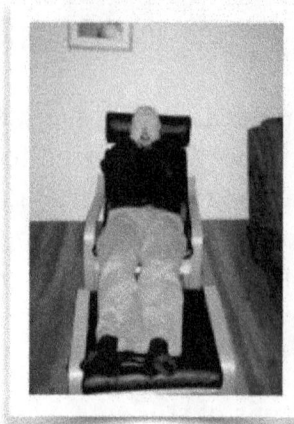
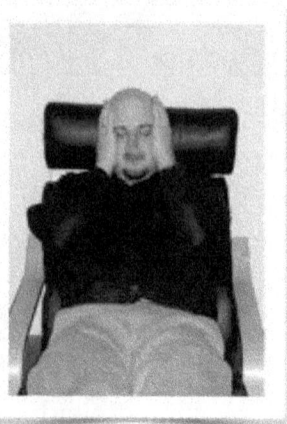
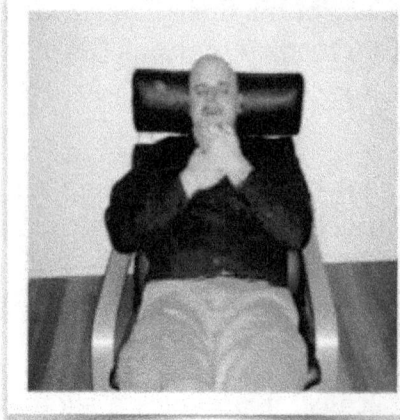
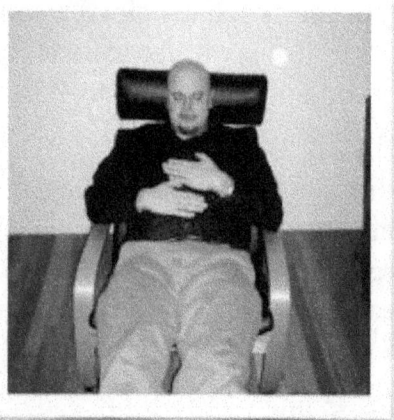
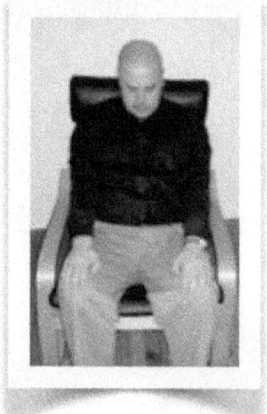

Self-Soothing Hands (SSH): The Method

1. Put your hands in front of you. Imagine you are holding the spirit of someone to whom you are deeply grateful between your hands.

2. Envision an endless supply of pure love, peace, comfort and good feeling coming out of the universe, through the top of your head, and flowing down your arms into your hand. Channel those pure feelings toward the spirit you are envisioning holding between your hands. Let it flow for a minute. You may feel your hands warm up or tingle slightly.

3. Move your hands up to cover your eyes, with your fingers themselves covering the front of your forehead. Breathe in compassion for yourself, and let the energy flow. You should feel the warm or tingling energy wax, then wane. All the while, reflect on the things for which you are grateful.

4. Move your hands to the sides of the face, to hold your own cheeks. Let the warmth/tingling feeling wax and wane as you again think grateful thoughts.

5. Put one hand over your neck and the other hand over your upper chest. Again, think grateful thoughts and allow the love/peace/comfort energy flow through you, waxing and waning.

6. Allow your two hands to cover your solar plexus region. Allow the gratitude thoughts to continue, and experience the waxing and waning of the energy.

7. Allow your two hands to rest on your lower abdomen. Allow the love/comfort/peace energy to flow through your hands to that center of worry and stress. When you feel it resolve, move on.

8. Finally, put both of your hands on your knees. Allow the energy to flow. Reflect on your grateful thoughts. Sense the movement of the comfort/peace/love energy as it moves through your knees and legs. Allow it to resolve, and then rest.

The tradition states that the "energy flows where it needs to go." You do not direct this energy. You just allow it to turn on and off. As such, you can not "Reiki" anyone except to become a conduit for this peaceful energy, but you can share it with those whom you love.

For more information on this technique, you may be interested in the book *Reiki Psychology*, which is currently available in various formats at online bookstores.

Applications of Self-Soothing Hands (SSH)

The nice thing about this technique is that you can utilize it, fully or partially, anytime you want to do so. You can even do it inconspicuously — for instance, in a meeting — by simply resting your hands on your legs or folded on your abdomen.

This technique is a great stress reliever for the following conditions:

- Mild to acute worry
- Feelings of sadness
- Various forms of daily stress
- Various body discomforts
- Insomnia
- Muscle tension
- Angry feelings

As gratitude is incompatible with hostility, this is a wonderful daily practice for someone who is frequently irritated or angry, or someone who just needs to calm down a little bit.

You can also use this practice directly with your loved ones. Channel the feelings of gratitude and the loving/soothing/peaceful energy when you are working with your children or your pets to see how they respond. You may find you are able to cultivate a calming "frequency" or "vibration" for yourself, which soothes the child or pet as well.

The more you practice this, the more dramatic your results will be.

Chapter 9: Gratitude Tapping (GT)

Note: I believe the 1MinuteHealing.com system is complete and effective. I am including other healing systems I use in my practice in these sections of the book in order to offer an expanded understanding of the concepts that have been woven into the PAWS system.

A wonderful tool that you should look up on the Internet (YouTube is fine) is called the Emotional Freedom Technique, or EFT. This was developed decades ago by man named Gary Craig, and professional certifications in the technique are only recently being offered.

The beauty in the technique is that it serves as quick way to resolve very strong feelings, and has been shown to be effective in the treatment of trauma. It falls into a class of therapies known as the "somatic" therapies, simply meaning that it is a body-based technique for the resolution of long-term or "stuck" feeling states.

The technique is amazingly simple to learn and apply. I have used it daily for years myself and I utilize it in my sessions with clients. However, there is an important thing that I believe is missing from EFT, and so I am writing about adding that here.

Typical EFT

In traditional EFT, you start by determining what number, from 0 to 10, you are going to "rate" the feeling created by a problem. This is called "Subjective Units of Distress" or the SUDs level. So for example, I might rate my feelings of anger toward a coworker as a 7, because she spread rumors about me. So in my head I rate the statement "I am angry because she spread rumors" as a 7 out of 10.

The next step is locating the sore spot or tapping the "karate chop" point of one of your hands. If you locate the sore spot, which rests about an inch under your collarbone, somewhere along its line, you rub it in a circle and repeat the following affirmation three times. If choose the "karate chop" point of your hand, you simply tap it with the four fingers of your opposite hand and state the following:

Say: "Even though I have [this problem], I deeply and completely accept myself."

So in my example it would be: "Even though *I am angry because my coworker spread rumors*, I deeply and completely accept myself."

This is to set up an important cognitive dissonance. Usually, when we have a problem, we blame ourselves for having the problem (even if we believe the problem originated with someone else, as in this example). By tapping or rubbing in a circle and making that accepting statement, you are short-circuiting the process of blaming yourself for having a problem and the resulting bad feelings.

The next steps of EFT involve simply stating the problem as a short phrase while tapping various points quickly with two fingers of one of your hands.

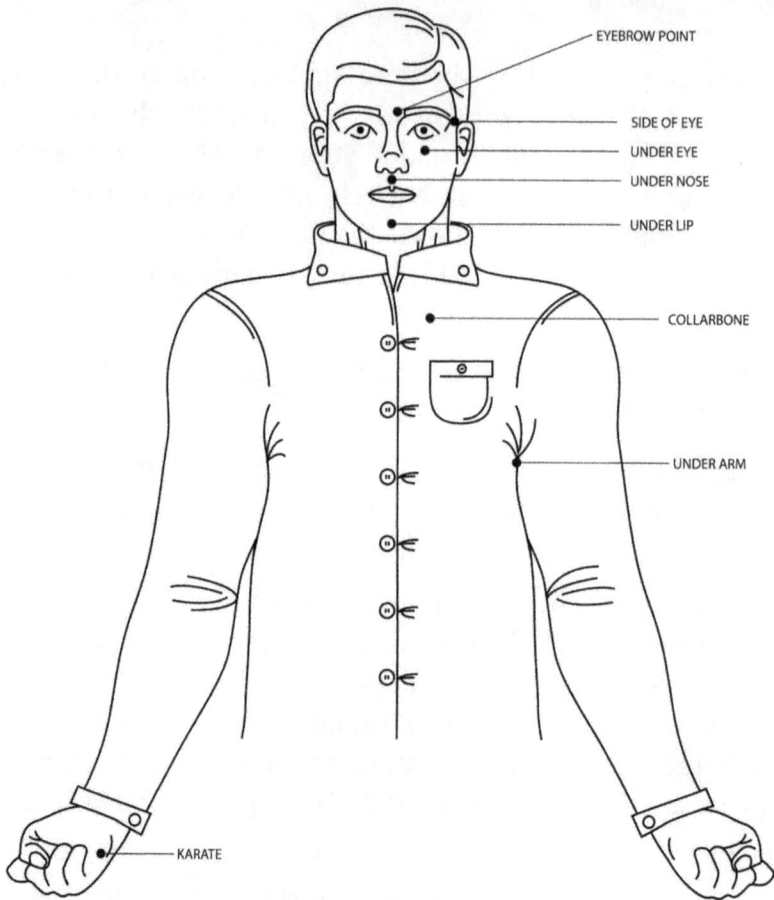

Labels on figure:
EYEBROW POINT
SIDE OF EYE
UNDER EYE
UNDER NOSE
UNDER LIP
COLLARBONE
UNDER ARM
KARATE

1. Inner Eyebrow (IE) on one side

2. Side of the Eye (SE), level with the pupil, on the bone

3. Under the Eye (UE), even with the pupil, on the bone

4. Under the Nose (UN)

5. Under the Lip (UL)

6. Collarbone (CB)

7. Under the Arm (UA)

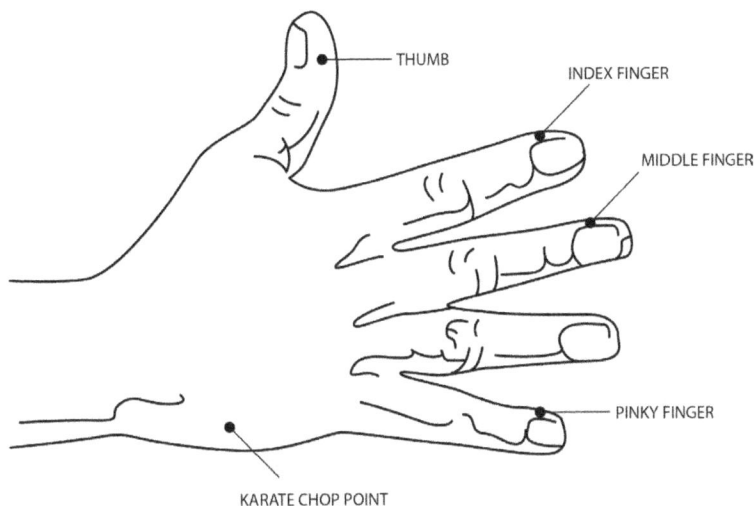

THUMB

INDEX FINGER

MIDDLE FINGER

PINKY FINGER

KARATE CHOP POINT

8. Side of the Thumb's nail bed (T) (tapping with opposite hand)

9. Side of the Index Finger's nail bed (IF)

10. Side of the Second Finger's nail bed (SF)

11. Side of the Pinky's nail bed (PF) (skipping the ring finger)

12. Karate Chop point of the hand (KC) (tapping with four fingers)

For each tapping point, going along with the previous example, I might say a few times to myself, "*Angry she spread rumors about me*" while I am tapping.

Following that, there is an optional "9-Gamut Procedure" which involves some eye movements, humming, and counting, all of which I am not going to go into here. There are really great videos on YouTube, though, and I urge you to check them out.

At the end of the procedure, you take inventory of your SUDs level, or how you feel. So for me, if my SUDs was at 7 when I started, it is likely to be a 2 or even a 1 by the time I stop. Gary Craig advises either continuing to tap until it gets down to 0, or finding a different facet (aspects) of the problem that may be unresolved and upsetting, and tapping on those, until the whole problem is down to 0.

In a way, it can be considered an "ordeal treatment" which exhausts the client into not having the problem, but it is much more than that. Research has shown this technique can reduce cortisol levels 20 percent for each round of tapping, and therefore, it is thought to break the association between the thought and the stress hormone cortisol.

Why change a good thing?

I did not make changes to this technique because I believe EFT is ineffective. In fact, I regard it as one of the most effective techniques and it is gaining research acceptance. I modified it simply because I think if we add gratitude to the practice, it will work better.

It is like having a favorite spice. Some people put their favorite spice on nearly everything because it enhances the flavor. For me, the most effective mental health tool is gratitude, so I think gratitude can be combined with EFT to make it that much better.

Gratitude Tapping (GT)

Just like with EFT, you identify your subjective units of distress, or SUDs level. You need a distressful feeling and a distressful thought. So "[Feeling] that [thought]." My example was "*Angry that coworker spread rumors.*" My SUDs level might be 7 out of 10.

In Gratitude Tapping (GT), you start with an affirmation while tapping the Karate Chop (KC) point: "Even though I have [this problem], I am deeply in my heart grateful that I have [this asset or resource]." In GT, you do not use the sore spot as you may in EFT, because the sore spot actually hurts.

You avoid self-violence of any kind in Gratitude-Based Techniques (GBT), a principle called *ahimsa*, Sanskrit for "to not injure" and foundational to many eastern religions such as Buddhism, Hinduism, and Jainism. The thought is that any injury to the self is also injury to all creatures, and vice-versa. That is why we do not use the sore spot in Gratitude Tapping, but rather, the Karate Chop (KC) point.

So in my example, it would be "Even though *I'm angry my coworker spread rumors*, I am deeply in my heart grateful that I have *the ability to calm down now and discuss my concerns with her.*" This is said while tapping the Karate Chop point on one hand with the four fingers of the other hand.

The next step is to tap each point while stating both the exposure statement *("Angry that coworker spread rumors")* <u>followed by</u> the gratitude statement *("grateful I can calm down and talk to her")*. The point of doing this is to use the neutralizing and calming power of gratitude in addition to the cortisol drop delivered by the tapping.

The use of humor

I have observed with hundreds of clients that one or two passes of Gratitude Tapping completely eliminates the need for the 9-Gamut procedure, especially if you use humor for the gratitude part of the statement. Humor is an incredibly robust psychological defense.

In the above scenario, I would suggest:

"Even though *I'm angry my coworker spread rumors*, I am deeply in my heart grateful that *I can leave her at the office to get coffee.*"

That is not just (maybe very) slightly humorous, but it indicates something for which one may be truly grateful: the ability to get coffee. The ability to confer a benefit (coffee) upon oneself, and thereby self-soothe, is very powerful. In fact, in my experience it is the people who are constantly dosing themselves on the "good things in life" who have better lives, in general.

Simple behavioral math for gratitude

It is simple, behavioral math. If you want life to be happier, have more happy things than sad things. If you don't have as many happy things as you would like, it is your responsibility (and no one else's) to create them. If for some reason you cannot have what you want, it is your responsibility to pick something else attainable and pursue that thing, instead of the first thing you wanted.

Be grateful for what you have, and add more numerous good things. Then use those things you gain in your gratitude procedures.

You have just learned *feeling better*, presented as a formula.

Chapter 10: Other healing modalities

This is a brief discussion of the types of things I frequently use in psychotherapy with my clients. These consulting techniques are most effective in the presence of a qualified, licensed mental health professional. I believe that the things in this section need to be handled in a consulting room to provide the customization, professional care, and privacy that only an in-person session with a qualified person can provide to you.

For Trauma: Somatic Experiencing, EFT, EMDR, and EMI

There are two kinds of trauma.

One is the kind everyone thinks about: *acute trauma.* Car accidents, various kinds of abuse, near death experiences, the horrors of war, witnessing tragic deaths, suddenly losing functioning are all on that list.

The second form is a kind of trauma that not a lot of people think about, and it is sometimes called *developmental trauma.* This is the trauma that occurs to our systems when life is difficult, and everyone has things that get us into a funk. Developmental trauma may occur over a much longer period of time than acute trauma.

The modern tools for developmental and acute trauma are the same. The good news is that they can also be used for temporary emotional upset. As stated before, my absolute favorite is the Emotional Freedom Technique (EFT) developed by Gary Craig. Research has demonstrated that cortisol levels drop when using acupoint tapping techniques such as EFT. My modification (GT) includes gratitude.

EFT and GT access acupressure points associated with calm while performing an exposure to a stimulus that is emotionally and mentally painful. A skilled interviewer is needed for a really good EFT/GT session, and that is why while I highly recommend the videos available for EFT/GT, they are not sufficient, and *especially for acute trauma*. I strongly recommend therapy sessions for those with acute trauma. The EFT/GT in those cases should only be practiced by someone who really excels in his or her interviewing skills and has a license to practice mental health techniques in the place it is done.

Somatic therapies such as Somatic Experiencing by Peter Levine, EFT by Gary Craig, Eye Movement Desensitization and Reprocessing (EMDR) by Francine Shapiro, Thought Field Therapy (TFT) by Roger Callahan, and Eye Movement Integration Therapy (EMI) out of the neurolinguistic programming movement all address trauma of various kinds faster and more effectively than talk therapy.

Here's a basic way to identify trauma: If something deeply bothers you, for a really long time, it is probably trauma-based rather than a problem that can be resolved using talk therapy alone. You can practice your way out of a trauma pattern using cognitive techniques, but using a somatic therapy (or several) will take much less time, because somatic therapies access the older, deeper brain level of trauma.

In my practice, I use GT and EMI. I learned EFT years ago in a training, and I have a certification in EMI. The other therapies mentioned are very effective as well, and I am open to learning and experiencing them. I have had some EMDR myself with great success.

For Coping, Behavior Change & Panic Attacks: Clinical Hypnosis

Clinical hypnosis is now used around the world for behavioral rehearsals. It is performed with Olympic-level athletes to enhance performance. We know from brain videos that the very same parts of the brain that would carry out a behavior in real life are working under hypnosis. So it is reasonable to use hypnosis to install a new behavior pattern, or rehearse a specific kind of performance.

The beauty of hypnosis is that a behavior pattern can be re-hearsed several times, very rapidly. The new behavior pattern can also be paired with mastery states evoked in the consulting room — feeling really good, confident, competent and success-ful. The athlete, for example, can master a new maneuver multiple times, and more rapidly than possible in a live rehears-al. The nascent public speaker can give a speech while feeling mastery states to various audiences, in the space of one hypno-sis session.

For coping, hypnosis can also be a wonderful tool. It is possible to hypnotically travel back in time to a trauma, distort it by inserting a mastery state, and then have "future rehearsals" of that situation with the accompanying mastery state.

Dealing with a non-preferred habit can be rehearsed out under hypnosis and accompanying tools from a discipline called neurolinguistic programming (NLP). Frequent requests in my practice are changing eating patterns, developing an exercise routine, and quitting smoking.

Finally, hypnosis is a wonderful accompanying treatment for cognitive behavioral therapy for panic attacks. The necessary exposures can be done under hypnosis, reducing the need to perform those exposures in "real life." This can shorten the duration of the treatment.

Influence and Clear Thinking: Neurolinguistic Programming

Neurolinguistic programming (NLP) has been widely used as a consulting tool for influence. Its origins are in the hypnotic work of Dr. Milton H. Erickson and the study of effective psychothera-pists such as Virginia Satir and Fritz Perls. It has been used in everything from psychotherapy to advertising. It is much-maligned as a psychotherapeutic technique because its early claims were too broad, as were the claims of other various therapies when they were developed. It is, however, a wonderful way to clarify one's thinking and dispel problematic ideas when combined with a similar therapeutic modality like one of the cognitive behavioral therapies.

After my certification in the technique, I was able to draw out my most significant learnings and apply them in psychotherapy. Among the best are:

1. Most people under-explain what they mean when they communicate. There is a principle widely discussed in NLP, borrowed from Alfred Korzybski, a Polish philosopher and scientist, that states "The map is not the territory." The way people represent thoughts to themselves is not the essence of reality. That is why it is useful to tell people that all thoughts are fictions, and that they have a choice in how they will represent reality to themselves. This is one of my favorite challenges to the way people think: "Is that a useful or non-useful fiction?"

2. Most people "scrunch up time." They believe that the past dictates what happens in the present, and the present dictates what will happen in the future. Therefore, by the transitive property, the past is the future. This is absolutely false (though we do know that without a meaningful behavioral intervention, past behavior is a pretty reliable predictor of future behavior). The goal in psychotherapy harnessing the power of things like mindfulness and NLP is to teach people that the past is not the future, and in fact, anything can happen at any time to radically alter a person's situation. This moment can be harnessed for powerful and lasting change. The hope in NLP is that the client will learn to independently act on a revised mental map of a situation right now, rather than waiting for the external reality to change by itself.

3. Brief change is possible utilizing the underutilized tools given to us by our neurology. All we have to do, using NLP techniques, is closely monitor the way a person represents something in order to harness the power of changing it. A combination of making good verbal contracts, changing eye movements, altering language, using imagination, and shifting affective responses can bring about dramatic change in a short amount of time.

For Managing Stress & Pain, Enhancing Well-Being: Self-Reiki

To master the comforting power of positive states, a person can learn the Japanese hands-on energy healing technique Reiki for lowering stress, increasing relaxation, and ultimately managing chronic pain.

I do not perform Reiki on anyone in my sessions, despite my training. Instead, I take a few non-traditional shortcuts and teach the person sitting in the consulting room how to perform it for oneself. In fact, I have a video on YouTube with a large number of views called "Learn Reiki in 10 Minutes." I also wrote a small book a few years ago titled *Reiki Psychology.*

I strongly believe in people having a large toolbox of techniques that they can use for themselves. Reiki is a technique, similar to meditation, that straddles good psychotherapeutic practice and spirituality. I believe as our practice of psychology advances, we will be incorporating more somatic and energy therapies, particularly as they are shown to be effective at achieving measurable health outcomes.

Chapter 11: The Research

The following essays share information supporting the techniques utilized in this skills manual.

Gratitude and its effects on well-being

In addition to my own aforementioned research, several studies have been conducted and theories have been postulated indicating that people who list what they are thankful for, on a regular basis, experience a higher sense of psychological well-being than those who do not engage in this practice.

According to Emmons and McCullough (2003), the findings from their studies indicate that groups of participants who practiced "counting their blessings versus burdens," exhibited a higher sense of well-being. Emmons and McCullough (2003) propose that Fredrickson's (1998, 2000) "broaden and build model of positive emotions" is a plausible explanation for these findings. Fredrickson wrote that positive emotions can aid in broadening an individual's mindset and build endearing personal relationships (Fredrickson, 1998) which, in return, can be used as additional resources during difficult times. Based on this model, Emmons and McCullough (2003) posit that gratitude, classified as a positive emotion, could be instrumental in helping people develop positive psychological, social, and spiritual resources that, in turn, elevate a person's sense of well-being.

Concluding findings from Lin and Yeh's (2013) study on the relationship among gratitude, social support, coping style, and well-being support the notion that as people continue to experience the positive benefits of expressing and embracing gratitude as a way of life, there is a significant increase in the development of coping skills, social connectedness, and overall psychological well-being. The benefits from practicing gratitude may lead to forming healthy friendships in which the person who expresses gratitude experiences a sense of contentment and thankfulness, and the recipient feels valued and appreciated. Thus, during difficult times, the individual feels a sense of reassurance and security in recalling what she is grateful for and knowing that she has support from her friends. Additionally, religions that incorporate the importance of gratitude help people develop a positive outlook on life and other people.

In Nelson's (2009) review entitled, "Can gratitude be used as a psychological intervention to improve individual well-being?" she states that clients who implement gratitude as part of psychotherapeutic interventions experience a higher sense of psychological well-being, based on the positive outcomes the individual experiences as a result. Based on the direction of the research thus far, a conclusion can firmly be drawn to support that the act of gratitude helps people focus on the positive rather than the negative aspects of their lives, which results in forming positive social connections, developing an overall positive outlook during challenging times, and a perhaps subjectively, a stronger spiritual connection to themselves and others.

Benefits of mindfulness meditation

Mindfulness meditation has been gaining momentum among psychologists as a method for aiding individuals in reducing cortisol levels which result in developing a healthier life style, lower levels of stress, and an overall sense of well-being. High levels of cortisol contribute to an individual feeling more anxious, depressed, and helpless. By contrast, reduced cortisol levels are noted in helping people feeling calm and confident in being able to work through difficult situations. This is a notable benefit.

Butler (2007) postulated in his dissertation that the application of mindfulness meditation aided in study participants being able to identify and accept their feels in a given situation and find the courage to navigate through challenging times. The participants indicated that they felt more courageous; however, this did not imply that they did not experience feelings of fear. The acceptance of feelings, whether they be negative or positive, helped the participants cope with the intense feelings that are usually accompanied by the circumstances they were facing.

Malcoun (2009) conducted a study entitled the *Psychological processes underlying the health benefits of a mindfulness-based stress reduction program.* The purpose of the study was to show the impact of this technique on the individual's "mindfulness, psychological symptoms, and physical functions." After the eight-week study, some participants indicated positive benefits.

The effects of mindfulness meditation upon the regulation of the neuroendocrine system were examined in a collaborative pilot study facilitated by Manzaneque et al (2011) in an article entitled "Psychobiological Modulation In Anxious And Depressed Patients After A Mindfulness Meditation Programme." According to their findings, participants who practiced mindfulness meditation showed improvement in lowering and regulating cortisol levels, which are correlated with the participant being able to better modulate the neuroendocrine system. These findings were obtained through blood sampling and providing participants with pre- and post-tests. Participants in the mindfulness condition showed an overall greater sense of well-being.

Benefits of compassion (Metta) meditation

There is no doubt that meditation can contribute to a sense of well-being for many people. Many of those who engage in this practice have reported that they have gained a better ability to focus and maintain a higher awareness of their surroundings, which helps them to be fully present in the "here and now." The next wave in this research is looking at the exercise of compassionate meditation.

Baer, Lykins, and Peters (2013) collected psychological data from experienced meditators to determine the characteristics common to meditators. Even though the study did not include information on the various types of meditation techniques the participants engage in, the outcome, overall, shows that self-compassion and mindfulness are strong indicators of well-being. In fact, the authors found that self-compassion was a better predictor of psychological well-being than mindfulness practice.

The purpose of a study conducted by Kemeny et al (2012) was to determine if non-religious practices could also be an influencing factor in boosting positive emotions and prosocial behavior. The focus was on the implementation of the secular version of meditation in providing similar outcomes to the religious practice of the same. According to their findings, individuals who are taught the practice of meditating and who exercise this technique on a regular basis are more apt to experience positive thoughts and emotions that lead to the reduction of negative thought processes. Once the negative thoughts are reduced, individuals are less likely to experience negative and unpleasant emotion. Furthermore, once these emotions are decreased, the individual is less likely to act upon any remaining negative thought processes.

Galante et al (2014) examined the findings from 22 studies that were geared toward finding conclusive evidence to support the hypothesis that kindness-based meditation, as opposed to the standard mindfulness forms of meditation, can significantly increase an individual's sense of well-being. The fundamentals of this hypothesis are based on previous studies indicating that meditation has a positive impact on the degree of kindness toward self and others; therefore, the implementation of kindness with meditation was believed to be a more effective intervention in the development of psychological well-being. Findings suggest that kindness-based meditation may benefit individuals and communities via effects on well-being and social interaction.

Research supporting EFT

Psychotherapy has been slowly progressing toward accepting the notion that techniques originating from Eastern Medicine positively influence the human psyche. The technique of stimulating an individual's acupoints, in particular, has gained a lot of momentum in the United States. Many people have reported that acupuncture and acupressure have been instrumental in helping resolve difficult psychological issues. The techniques that have emerged chiefly from people who have ties to neuro-linguistic programming (NLP) are acupoint tapping such as the Emotional Freedom Techniques (EFT) and Eye Movement Desensitization and Reprocessing (EMDR).

Previous studies and reports from clients have indicated that the incorporation of EFT/acupoint tapping in their therapy session have produced significant positive results in being able to process and manage trauma and anxiety. One of the most commonly known disorders that has proven to be successfully treated by the utilization of these techniques is Post Traumatic Stress Disorder (Feinstein, 2012). Feinstein was able to show, in his meta-analysis of 51 peer-reviewed papers and 18 random-ized controlled clinical trials, that several studies have pointed to the efficacy of acupoint tapping in resolving long-term emo-tional problems.

In a study conducted by Church (2010), the Emotional Freedom Techniques, as compared to other therapeutic interventions, produced better outcomes in treating combat veterans with PTSD than traditional therapies. The study suggests the imple-mentation of acupoint stimulation techniques while recalling and activating memories surrounding a highly aversive event produce the desired results in altering the client's neurochemis-try associated with that experience. Church also indicates that blood cortisol levels were lower in clients who received just one hour-long session of EFT.

The combination of a sense of empowerment and lowered cortisol levels apparently results in the client's ability to manage future unpleasant circumstances. Emotional Freedom Tech-niques focus on the client's ability to have the freedom to choose how they perceive unpleasant circumstances, which contributes to providing clients with the awareness that they are capable of changing how they feel about these circumstances.

Emerging directions in Reiki research

In the past several decades, Reiki has gained popularity among healthcare professionals in hospital and hospice settings in the United States. The fundamental premise of Reiki is the application of a subtle, relaxing, healing energy. Applying Reiki techniques are usually performed by the professional placing their hands on the parts of the body that correspond with the patient's endocrine and lymph systems (LaTorre, 2005). Initially, the practitioner must undergo training before being able to practice Reiki and teach it to their clients.

Clients can be taught to perform Reiki when they are experiencing emotional discomfort. Incorporating Reiki into a therapy session can enhance the interpersonal relationship between therapist and client as well as provide the client with a sense of empowerment. A client can learn to use this technique, outside of the therapy session, to bring about a sense of inner peace when it is needed. Numerous clients who regularly experience stress, anxiety, depression, or chronic pain, report that the application of Reiki has been successful in reducing this issues (La Torre, 2005).

The evidence is building. Scholarly research includes the following.

- In one study of advanced cancer patients, the participants who received Reiki treatments in addition to their pain medication experienced improvements in pain control and reported quality of life (Olson, Hanson, & Michaud; 2005).

- Relief from pain and anxiety was reported in women who received three 30-minute sessions of Reiki after abdominal hysterectomy. They reported less pain and requested fewer pain medication administrations (Vitale & O'Connor, 2006).

- Older adults who received a 30-minute Reiki treatment weekly for eight weeks reported significant decreases in symptoms of anxiety, depression, and pain compared to those receiving no treatment (Richeson, Spross, Lutz, & Peng; 2010).

- Reiki may help men experience less anxiety when being treated with external beam radiotherapy for prostate cancer (Beard et al, 2010).

- Highly significant pain reduction was reported after Reiki treatments for a variety of pain-related conditions, including cancer, in a study of 20 people experiencing pain at 55 locations. (Olson & Hanson, 1997).

There are many more sources available that offer summaries of the positive effects of Reiki, but this list constitutes a starting point showing its apparent efficacy for psychological factors related to pain, depression, anxiety, and well-being.

Research on Clinical and Self-Hypnosis

Clinical hypnotherapy is commonly incorporated into the work of psychotherapy. There have been numerous studies and articles published in refereed journals which provide substantial results as to the efficacy of using clinical hypnosis in treat patients with psychological disorders (Lynn et al, 1996).

Clinicians have been successful in sorting out what clinical hypnosis is and is not. First of all, clinical hypnosis is not a trance or altered state of consciousness activated by a hypnotist. Rather, the effectiveness of hypnosis hinges upon the client's efforts and abilities to do that (Lynn et al, 2014). Second, hypnosis is not the act of imposing the hypnotist's will upon the one being hypnotized. The client has full control of their faculties, and they are capable of accepting or rejecting suggestions during the treatment process. Third, clinical hypnosis is not haphazardly practiced by untrained therapists. Practicing clinicians are required to receive training before they can use its applications in the therapeutic setting. Last, hypnosis is not only useful as a relaxation technique. It can also be used to enhance alertness and create behavioral rehearsals (Lynn et al, 2014).

There are many benefits to including hypnosis in the therapy session. It can be used as another form of personal and meaningful communication between therapist and client that may be difficult to accomplish with standard two-way conversation (Lynn et al, 2014). The therapist can introduce abstract concepts, metaphors, and ideas that represent real-life situations that might be challenging for the client to bring to the surface. This can be especially helpful with children who have undergone a traumatic experience. Clients may find hypnosis as a beneficial way of imagining alternate scenarios. For example, hypnosis could be used in conjunction with the Solution Focused Therapy's "Miracle Question." Likewise, the flexible nature of hypnosis enables it to work well with various psychotherapeutic theories and treatment techniques.

There is a vast amount of research supporting the efficacy of hypnosis for various beneficial outcomes. Here is an abbreviated list.

- Twenty-one patients received three sessions of hypnosis for smoking cessation. At the end of treatment 81% reported they quit smoking, and 48% reported abstinence at 12 month followup (Elkins & Rajab, 2004)

- Twice the number of smokers who quit using hypnosis stayed smoke-free at two year follow-up, compared to those who quit without hypnosis, in a study of 71 participants (Wynd, 2005).

- Hypnotherapy resulted in an average of 17 pounds of weight loss at six-month followup in a study of 60 women who started the study 20% overweight, compared to a control group that did not receive hypnotherapy. (Cochrane & Friesen, 1986).

- In a study of 61 burn patients, those with high baseline pain reported greater relief from hypnosis than high-baseline-pain controls who did not receive hypnosis (Patterson & Ptacek, 1997).

- In a study of 261 veterans admitted to the Substance Abuse Residential Rehabilitation Treatment Programs (SARRTPs), those who used self-hypnosis at least 3-5 times per week reported the highest levels of self-esteem and serenity, and the least anger and impulsivity, in comparison to minimal-practice and control groups. (Pekala et al, 2004).

Thus, the effects of clinical hypnosis and self-hypnosis for retraining the brain to achieve better behavioral outcomes appears to be well-documented in the scientific literature.

References

Baer, R. A., Lykins, E. B., & Peters, J. R. (2012). Mindfulness and self-compassion as predictors of psychological wellbeing in long-term meditators and matched nonmeditators. *The Journal Of Positive Psychology, 7*(3), 230-238. Doi: 10.1080/ 17439760.2012.674548

Beard, C., Stason, W. B., Wang, Q., Manola, J., Dean-Clower, E., Dusek, J. A., DeCristofaro, S., Webster, A., Doherty-Gilman, A. M., Rosenthal, D. S., & Benson, H. (2010). Effects of com plementary therapies on clinical outcomes in patients being treated with radiation therapy for prostate cancer. *Cancer, 117*(1), 96-102.

Butler, M. M. (2007). *The experience of mindfulness meditation as learned in a brief, structured mindfulness meditation course: A qualitative investigation.* (Order No. 3276695, The University of Memphis). *ProQuest Dissertations and Theses,* 104. Retrieved from http://search.proquest.com/docview/304717506?accountid=4488. (304717506).

Church, D. (2010). The treatment of combat trauma in veterans using EFT (Emotional Freedom Techniques): A pilot protocol. *Traumatology, 16*(1), 55-65. doi:10.1177/1534765609347549

Cochrane, G., & Friesen, J. (1986). Hypnotherapy in weight loss management. *Journal of Consulting and Clinical Psychology, 54,* 489-492.

Emmons, R., & McCullough, M. (2003). Counting Blessings Versus Burdens: An Experimental Investigation Of Gratitude And Subjective Well-being In Daily Life. *Journal of Personality & Social Psychology,* 377-389.

Elkins, G. R. & Rajab, M. H. (2004). Clinical hypnosis for smoking cessation: preliminary results of a three-session intervention. *Int J Clin Exp Hypn, 52*(1), 73-81.

Feinstein, D. (2012). Acupoint stimulation in treating psychological disorders: Evidence of efficacy. *Review Of General Psychology, 16*(4), 364-380. doi:10.1037/a0028602

Galante, J., Galante, I., Bekkers, M., & Gallacher, J. (2014). Effect of Kindness-Based Meditation on Health and Well-Being: A Systematic Review and Meta-Analysis. *Journal Of Consulting and Clinical Psychology,* doi:10.1037/a0037249

Kemeny, M. E., Foltz, C., Cavanagh, J. F., Cullen, M., Giese-Davis, J., Jennings, P., &... Ekman, P. (2012). Contemplative/emotion training reduces negative emotional behavior and promotes prosocial responses. *Emotion,* 12(2), 338-350. doi:10.1037/a0026118

LaTorre, M. A. (2005). The use of Reiki in psychotherapy. *Perspectives In Psychiatric Care, 41*(4), 184-187. doi:10.1111/j.1744-6163.2005.00035.

Lin, C., & Yeh, Y. (2013). How Gratitude Influences Well-Being: A Structural Equation Modeling Approach. *Social Indicators Research.* Retrieved November 13, 2014.

Lynn, S. J., Kirsch, I., Neufeld, J., & Rhue, J. W. (1996). Clinical Hypnosis: Assessment, Applications, and Treatment Considerations. In S. J. Lynn, I. Kirsch, J. W. Rhue (Eds.), *Casebook of clinical hypnosis* (pp. 3-30). Washington, DC, US: American Psychological Association. doi:10.1037/11090-001

Lynn, S. J., Woody, E. Z., Montgomery, G., & Gaudiano, B. (2014). Hypnosis: Contributions to psychological science and clinical practice. *Psychology Of Consciousness: Theory, Research, And Practice, 1*(2), 103-104. doi:10.1037/cns0000020

Malcoun, E. (2009). Unpacking mindfulness: Psychological processes underlying the health benefits of a mindfulness-based stress reduction program. *Dissertation Abstracts International: Sec tion B: The Sciences and Engineering, 69*(12-B), 7817-7817.

Manzaneque, J., Vera, F., Ramos, N., Godoy, Y., Rodriguez, F., Blanca, M.,... Enguix, A. (2011). Psychobiological Modulation In Anxious And Depressed Patients After A Mindfulness Meditation Programme: A Pilot Study. *Stress and Health,* 216-222.

Nelson, C. (2009). Appreciating gratitude: Can gratitude be used as a psychological intervention to improve individual well-being? *Counselling Psychology Review, 24*(3-4), 38-50.

Olson, K., & Hanson, J. (1997). Using Reiki to manage pain: a preliminary report. *Cancer Prevention & Control, 1*(2), 108-113.

Olson, K., Hanson, J., & Michaud, M. (2003). A phase II trial of Reiki for the management of pain in advanced cancer patients. *Journal of Pain and Symptom Management, 26*(5), 990-7.

Patterson, D. R., & Ptacek, J. T. (1997). Baseline pain as a moderator of hypnotic analgesia for burn injury treatment. *J Consult Clin Psychol, 65*(1), 60-7.

Pekala, R. J., Maurer, R. L., Kumar, V. K., Elliot, N. C., Masten, E., Moon E., et al. (2004). Self-hypnosis relapse prevention training with chronic drug/alcohol users: effects on self-esteem, affect, and relapse. *American Journal of Clinical Hypnosis, 46,* 281-97.

Richeson, N. E., Spross, J. A., Lutz, K., & Peng, C. (2010). Effects of Reiki on anxiety, depression, pain and physiological factors in community-dwelling older adults. *Research in Gerontological Nursing, 3*(3), 187-99.

Vitale, A.T., & O'Connor, P. C. (2006). The effect of Reiki on pain and anxiety in women with abdominal hysterectomies: a quasi-experimental pilot study. *Holistic Nursing Practice, 20*(6), 273-4.

Wynd, C. A. (2005). Guided health imagery for smoking cessation and long-term abstinence. *Journal of Nursing Scholarship, 37*(3), 245-250.

Chapter 12: A final word

Healing distinguishes itself by the boldest and most unapologetic form of love.

The contents of this guide either directly deliver love-as-healing, or create the space for love-as-healing to occur.

Love always was, always is, and always will be free. If you purchased this book, I am so grateful for your support of this work. If you obtained it for free, from a friend or me directly, know that I am honored you are even reading this.

Give it away. Show people what you have learned. It can only expand and enrich your life. It can only bring peace and hit to those around you, and that would be the highest good.

People can heal through anything, even the highest levels of performance. Don't underestimate the power of a healing to radically change the fortunes of yourself and everyone around you.

I am so grateful for you. Thank you for spreading healing into the world.

God bless.

R. Wolf Shipon
Lake Parsippany, NJ
June 1, 2016

About the Author

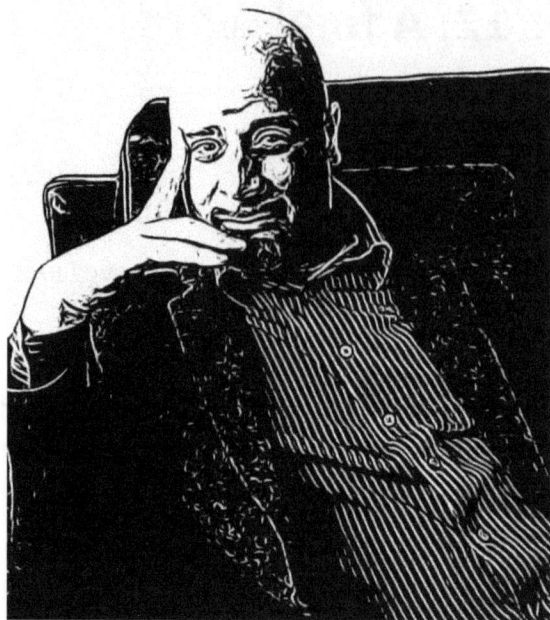

With a background in journalism and information technology, Dr. R. Wolf Shipon began his healing journey when he was misdiagnosed with Parkinson's Disease for 18 months in the late 1990s. In response to his befuddlement, he learned and then taught Reiki. He entered the field of mental health with a respect for alternative healing techniques. This passion has persisted through his various autoimmune disease diagnoses beginning in 2012.

His research into foundational healing ideas have laid the groundwork for three books on the topic, of which this is the latest as of 2016.

Dr. Shipon owns and operates a group psychotherapy practice in Mountain Lakes, NJ, (Inner Wellth LLC). He resides on a lake in Northern New Jersey with his wife, son, and two cats. He is an avid stand-up kayaker and ukulele player. His personal blog is at DrWolfShipon.com and features brief thoughts of the day based on his work and experiences.

www.ingramcontent.com/pod-product-compliance
Lightning Source LLC
Chambersburg PA
CBHW032119280326
41933CB00009B/907